...And now what do we do?

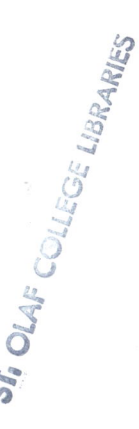

Published by EMMPS, Inc.
1203 South Maple Street, Northfield, MN 55057

All rights reserved. No part of this book may be reproduced or
transmitted in any form by any means, electronic or mechanical,
including photocopying, recording, or by any information storage
and retrieval system without written permission from the authors,
except for the inclusion of a brief quotation in a review.
Copyright Registration # 083559579
ISBN 0-9659200-0-3

©Robin and Loranelle Schroeder, 1996

. . .

For our mothers —

Evelyn Marie Mathilda Peterson Schroeder

&

Virginia Louisa Moore Tuttle

. . .

Table of Contents

Introduction	1
Chapter 1: And Now What Do We Do?	2
Chapter 2: Now We Know What's Available; Now What?	12
Chapter 3: The Facility & The Resident Services	22
Chapter 4: The Personnel	34
Chapter 5: Social Activities	44
Chapter 6: Family Services	52
Chapter 7: Costs, Funding and Legal Concerns	60
Chapter 8: Visiting the Facility	72
Chapter 9: Glossary	78
Chapter 10: Resources	86
Epilogue	97
Acknowledgments	98
Facility Evaluation Guide	

Introduction

The selection of a care facility for yourself or another family member is one of the most important choices you will make in your lifetime. There is as much to know about this process as there is about having and raising children or managing your own business or buying a house.

The difference is that there aren't many manuals or guides or handbooks or graduate programs to help you make the choice that is best for you. There is only you, aided in many cases by overworked social services professionals doing their best for you and their specific facilities.

There are three constants. At every turn you will discover 1) choices to be made, 2) challenges to be faced and 3) opportunities of which to take advantage.

The purpose of this handbook is to help you and your family define those choices, challenges and opportunities, then make logical, practical decisions. We are going to supply you with resource information, questions to ask, suggestions on whom to ask, and lists of things you can observe on your own. We hope you will take advantage of the format and make notes to yourself on the evaluation guide provided at the back of the book. Add your own questions, and make it a truly useful tool for you and your family.

There are two fundamental situations we are going to address. The first is a family's need to find a care facility for an aging or ill loved one. The second is a personal search for a facility for oneself. In either situation, the questions you need to ask and the answers you seek are the same. It's what gets you there that's different.

Throughout this handbook, we are also going to talk about the emotions accompanying these choices and share with you what we learned about our parents, ourselves and our friends. Neither of us is a trained psychologist or social services professional. We are simply people who were placed in a situation like so many others before us. To make sure that the information we included in this handbook is accurate, we have engaged professionals in these fields and within the health care industry to serve as our advisors.

We hope that telling our story will help other people live their stories. In fact, that's exactly where we are going to start.

1 And Now What Do We Do?

On Wednesday, March 15, 1995, we left the house to keep a business appointment. Robin's mother, who lived with us, remained home alone. We returned home about four hours later. As the garage door opened, all we could see was Mom sitting on the garage floor, her eyes as big as saucers. There was a cut above her left eye and blood on the garage floor. She was dazed and bewildered and had no idea how long she had been there. Lonnie called 911 as Robin comforted her. The paramedics arrived, examined her and took her to the hospital.

Robin went with his mother to the hospital and Lonnie stayed in our home office to keep an appointment. About two hours later, Robin called to say that Mom would be kept for observation. Lonnie took some clothes and personal things to the hospital. The three of us visited for awhile but Mom was exhausted and confused so we left. When we got home, Robin explained that the doctor had informed him Mom couldn't live with us anymore, that she needed twenty-four hour care we couldn't provide. He had also told Robin it was easier to admit a patient into a care facility from a hospital than from a private home. The doctor said he would help with the process as would the hospital social worker. Then he informed Robin that the hospital couldn't keep Mom over the weekend. She had to be released Friday.

If we were going to go this route, we had one day in which to find a suitable place for her.

And that's how this journey began.

When You Must Choose For A Loved One

To say we were distraught is an understatement. We were emotionally spent and completely at a loss. What we needed wasn't sleep, however. We needed information and we needed it now. We obviously had to make arrangements fast, and to do that we needed to overcome our emotional limbo and think speedily and efficiently about Mom's welfare.

There are so many levels of emotion in any decision involving people you love that it would be impossible to deal with them all. **Our best advice is to acknowledge whatever you are feeling.** To get past our own emotions that March afternoon, we needed to turn to each other, be honest and admit we were scared, panicked, guilty, sad, relieved, worried, angry and about a million other emotional adjectives. You get the idea. Once we acknowledged our emotions, we could draw strength from our mutual anxieties and were therefore able to plan our next couple of steps on a much more logical basis.

We talked about what we were feeling but also realized that we had to postpone dealing with those feelings. There was only one immediate priority: we needed to find a place for Mom. Later, when we talked about that initial realization, we almost felt lucky. Crisis can engender feelings that paralyze and immobilize. We knew we couldn't let that happen. We had to put our feelings on hold. Looking at the emotions later after they had partially subsided was somehow easier.

For example, each of us felt guilty that we were relieved Mom would be cared for by medical professionals outside of our home. We had been having a rough time with her erratic sleeping patterns and increased confusion. Not one of the three of us had been sleeping very well. Her

. . .

health was also failing much more rapidly than we had anticipated. It had been our responsibility to care for her, and we therefore wrongly concluded we had failed at the task. We had lost control. That couldn't be, could it?

We also felt guilty that our absence had somehow caused this accident. We still don't know why she was in the garage and it doesn't matter. Her story was never the same twice. It was, however, completely out of character for her to enter the garage for any reason other than to go somewhere with us. She was not inclined to leave the house at all. Nonetheless, we knew that if we had been home she would have been all right. That is reality; it is also reality that the inevitable would have only been delayed, not deterred. Among the best advice we received was the suggestion that we try to place our role in its proper perspective.

We felt a staggering anxiety that we would not find a decent facility and that she would somehow be worse off. Even though we live in a small town in a state known for exceptional health care, we were not sure we could find what we needed. We wanted desperately to do everything right, and we had just one day.

We needed support from our family. We are a very close-knit group and even though our family members are hundreds of miles away, we could feel their unconditional love when we called. It supplied us with a driving energy. However, we wasted a lot of time being upset that they weren't here and wishing they would arrive at any minute to help us. Now we can see that their physical presence wasn't important, and even realize it might have been an impediment. But we did not see it that way at the time. Nonetheless, what did count was their complete love, trust and affection, and the fact that they were constant sources of strength.

It is important to remember that siblings or other family members who live at a distance also need support. As the situation with an aging father or mother worsens, the anxieties of family members who are not involved in the day-to-day process increase dramatically. Every phone call becomes the call that could beckon them to help deal with the emergency, to drop everything and come. They struggle with the decision to go or stay, to deal with the guilt of their distance or the needs of their own families. Should they go on a vacation that they have planned for months? Should they take a leave from their jobs and come to help? What's best for them? For their siblings? For their aging parent? For their own family?

In our family, Robin and his brother, Don, worked through all the intricacies of these emotions very well. On several occasions, when Robin made what we referred to as the "tag-you're-it" call, Don came swiftly and willingly to help with whatever challenge was being faced. There are no martyrs or heroes or villains in this process. There is only your family and the needs of your loved one. Again, the honest expression of emotions and needs will be the best map to navigate this sea. Just remember that everyone has a unique set of concerns and issues with which they are dealing. Since there is nothing simple about any of these concerns, how could dealing with them be simple?

We were sad that Mom wouldn't be living with us anymore. Life with an aging parent isn't all hardship and strife. We had fun times, too. That they should end so abruptly was traumatic. What would happen to the jokes we shared at mealtime? Who would watch *The Lawrence Welk Show* with her?

We were worried Mom would fight this move tooth and nail. Fiercely independent, and personally private, Mom was not about to go to "a home" willingly. What would we do if she balked? Could we handle that? Of course, but did we want to? NO.

We were worried because Mom wasn't simply aging anymore. Now she was ill enough that we couldn't care for her. Did that mean she was dying? Could anyone care for her as well as we could? It was this emotion more than any other that spurred us to action.

Finally, we felt this was all unfair and unjust. Could we or should we have been more prepared? We had tried to do right by Robin's mother and now we felt punished. Why was this happening in this manner? What had we done to deserve it?

Of course, the answer was — nothing. Robin's mother was aging and ill. What happened had simply happened and now we had to deal with it. No blame was necessary and any more thought of blame would prove useless. This is when our time constraints really helped. We didn't have time for self pity or a soul searching analysis of God's will. We needed to act and we needed to act NOW.

That was our curse and our blessing.

When You Are Searching For Yourself

There are three primary circumstances that require you to select a care facility for yourself. One, you need to recuperate from surgery or require therapy for rehabilitation after, for example, a fall or broken bone. Two, you are ill, aging and need help. Three, you are planning ahead.

Since the first two are medically-related needs we urge you to begin by getting all the information you need from your physician. In the first case, what kind of therapy do you need? For how long? In the second, what needs do you have now and what needs will the future hold? Both of those answers will affect your choice. More information on what to ask your physician will follow in the next chapter.

The third scenario — care centers and our need for them — offers a picture of the best (and worst for some) of all possible worlds. Presumably, you are relatively healthy and trying to plan your future in such a manner that you will have a say in what ultimately happens. You can't predict your eventual medical needs, but you can find out what's available.

The emotions you need to deal with here will be directly related to how you deal with your own aging. Confronting the immediate emergency of dealing with Robin's mother, we began to consider our own future prospects. We have no children, and thought that meant we must plan much more extensively than would our friends whose children would care for them. We urge you not to fall into this "trap." First, having children doesn't guarantee you caregivers as you age. Second, why would you want to put your own children in this most difficult situation? Third, they may not understand your needs. **Give your family one of the greatest gifts you can and help to plan your own care. It is truly a loving thing to do.**

Among the best facilities we have found are those which combine a retirement center with a medical facility of some sort. In such a facility, you can live in the part of the complex that offers you independent living while you are able to do so. If your health degenerates, you can then move — within that same facility — to assisted living or to the medical care center. Some retirement centers even offer a hospital on the premises where more extensive health care needs can also be met.

Waiting lists are long at most places like this. Don't hesitate to put your names on the list. You can always decline if you aren't ready to make the move when your name reaches the top of the list. You will remain on the waiting list, and will then be able, without undue pressure, to continue analyzing your needs.

It can be disheartening and frightening to think of one's own aging and eventual need for concentrated health care. It can also be deeply comforting to know that you made those choices for yourself.

In either instance, find out what facilities are available in your area. Most hospitals have social services professionals who will help you locate facilities. County agencies may offer the same services. The beauty of having help from a professional is their knowledge of the facilities themselves. They may know people and they may be able to make appointments for you. No matter how you start, the decision is still going to wind up in your lap. Take what help you can get but never forget that one fact. Where does this buck stop? With you and you alone.

Your local church or community action center may also have help for you. Try the chamber of commerce too. There are many avenues to explore. Also, the Older Americans Act of 1975 requires every state to establish an ombudsman's office, which resolves complaints and advocates on behalf of nursing home residents. It can also supply basic information on the location of homes (or local ombudsman offices) in your area. The office for each state is listed in Chapter Ten.

There are many kinds of care facilities. The list which follows is meant to be general and to give you some basic parameters on what you might expect to find at each.

Non-Profit Organizations

Care Centers Affiliated with a Religion or Denomination: These facilities may offer special consideration to members of the denomination but usually do not require membership in that denomination to become a resident.

Care Centers Affiliated with an Organization: The Masons operate such facilities, as do the Odd Fellows. Check with the local chapter of these kinds of organizations and see if they have any information. Like facilities affiliated with a denomination, these centers usually do not require membership in their respective fraternal organization to become a resident. These organizations may also rely upon their membership to serve as volunteers who provide additional amenities, time or attention for their residents.

Unaffiliated Care Centers: Many non-profits need a guardian angel. For the types of care centers affiliated with a denomination, religion, or service organization the parent organization provides that help. If you are talking with an independent non-profit, find out how they support themselves. The center may be sponsored by a county or a city, thus drawing from their community for support and volunteers. Are their charges comparable to those of other affiliated facilities? Are families of the residents expected to help raise money? In other words, who is their guardian angel?

For-Profit Companies

As federal and state financial support becomes less reliable and as the number of elderly individuals grows, more and more companies see care centers as a profitable spin-off of the health care industry. From the outside, these facilities probably won't look different from those run by non-profits. Although they are in business to make money, you will still find caring professionals helping the residents. The questions you need to ask are the same no matter what the source of support.

There are also foster care homes that deal with fewer people. The size of the facility can be as small as two or three residents. We did not consider this as an option because of the number of well-respected care facilities in our area. Again, your county social services office should have information about this type of care.

Foster care homes can be "mom and pop" operations or corporate-sponsored homes, non-profit or for-profit facilities. The "mom and pop" variety homes provide a family-oriented atmosphere along with room and board. They are generally limited in the amount of assistance they can give the resident. Corporate adult foster care may enhance the family oriented room and board with staff who are able to cope with more behavior management problems or assist with more personal care.

Your timeline is irrelevant. Even if you are planning ahead you still need to know exactly what you must find to meet your loved one's needs. They may or may not be willing participants in this process. That must not in any way hinder your commitment to finding the right facility.

Understand what you are feeling and try to deal with it when you are able to deal with it. Exhaustion is not conducive to emotional well-being. Find somebody you can lean on when your fatigue level reaches "tilt." You really can get through this. Really.

> ### And now what do we do?
>
> - Acknowledge your emotions.
>
> - Place your role in its proper perspective.
>
> - Whether you are searching for a care center for you or a loved one, gather information on the facilities in your area. Use every resource available to you.
>
> - One of the greatest gifts you can give your family is to search out and select a care facility before you need one.

Now We Know What's Available; Now What?

We have compiled a list of the questions you need to ask any medical professional or facility you are considering. These questions can be asked over the phone or in person. There is, however, another list of things to look for on a visit to a care center.

Some of these questions are difficult because they can conjure up pictures of institutional warehousing for people who are already feeling remorse at the action they are taking for a loved one. Try to get past that and understand that if you don't ask these questions, you will not know what you or your loved one is getting into.

Where do we start?

First, you need to talk to the doctor. Our experience with medical professionals was wonderful. The overwhelming majority of the doctors, nurses, nurse practitioners, care technicians and therapists of all varieties who took care of Mom were dedicated people who did their jobs well. But these people speak their own language and you must find out what their words mean. **Be assertive. Get your answers.**

Questions to Ask Your Physician

1. *What medical problem(s) does your loved one have? Is this condition curable? What are the traits of the disease(s) or condition(s) and how will they affect (or have they affected) your loved one? What deterioration or ramifications of the disease(s) can you expect to see in the future? What treatment, if any, is available?*

It is still embarrassing to admit that neither of us realized dementia is a physical disease. Some of our erroneous assumptions about dementia made dealing with Mom on a day-to-day basis much harder than it really had to be. We thought she was "just forgetful." We thought she was angry at us when she was really angry at her inability to speak the right word or acclimate to her environment — to remember where she lived, to remember she was retired. When we finally starting asking the right questions we got the answers we needed.

We were also blessed with the physician who cared for Mom. She is a kind and sensitive soul who emotionally "held our hands" through this process. When she realized we didn't understand some of the information she had shared with us, she took extra time at our appointments and went out of her way to help us move Mom to a facility closer to our home which she visited regularly. She is also an advisor to us as we write this handbook. In short, she cares and proves it again and again.

We understand that our relationship with Mom's physician is not necessarily typical. We can only stress that you are the advocate for your loved one. Aggressive questioning and search for accurate information on their behalf is the most reasonable behavior you can exhibit. May each of you find a doctor like ours.

> 2. *What level of care does your loved one need? Round-the-clock? Daily visits by a nurse's aide? Help with personal hygiene? Help preparing meals? Help with medications?*

Asking about the medications was a crucial part of our final determination that we could no longer care for Mom. Compared with other

• • •

people her age (87), she didn't take many drugs, but she did have unusual and unpredictable reactions to some of them. For example, when we gave her a particular drug with codeine to soothe her after cataract surgery she became agitated and aggressive. We had to stay up with her all night just to prevent her from ripping the bandages from her eye.

As her health deteriorated, her needs increased, which in turn demanded increased attention and care from us. Soon we were in way over our heads. We began keeping charts and lists of all the pills and doses and times, etc. It was not impossible, but it was demanding. Also, we began to worry about how the medications were reacting with each other. That is a key consideration and a question which should be asked any time new medications are added.

If the physicians with whom you are dealing are unavailable, there are other good sources of information on medication. Check with the nursing staff or local pharmacy. There are also resource texts and software which explain things in common language. Contact any bookstore or software dealer for more information.

One of the most prevalent problems nursing staffs at care centers and family caregivers at home deal with is incontinence. This is a severe and debilitating problem for both the person suffering the indignity and the person caring for him or her. We learned that it was many times the "straw that broke the camel's back" for family caregivers. If your loved one suffers from this problem, try to understand that they are as embarrassed and humiliated as you are frustrated and angry. Each of these emotions is understandable and, like others we have discussed, shouldn't be ignored.

Mom was an extremely private person and did not want anyone helping her with personal hygiene. She refused in-home visits from aides because she didn't want to be on anyone's schedule other than her own. That significantly limited our care options. You may be thinking that we should have insisted on certain things. Perhaps so, but we believed at the time that for as long as she was mentally alert and emotionally and physically able, Mom had a right to make as many of the decisions about her own life as she could. That may have placed some extra burdens on us at times but the burdens seem slight when we consider how vulnerable she must have felt.

A vast amount of material has been written about the role-reversal which occurs between aging parents and their adult children. Everything we read — which didn't come close to being definitive — emphasized how difficult this was. Based on our experience, the authors are correct. Many of us have no choice but to jump into the emotional pool of parenting an aged parent and see if we can at least tread water. We found that the best thing we could do when we started floundering was to follow our hearts. As trite as this sounds, the love you feel for your family member is your emotional compass. We worked on this very simple premise: Robin's mother had our love and deserved our respect.

> 3. *What are your loved one's special medical needs? Physical therapy? Occupational therapy? Speech therapy? Why does he or she need these services? What is the prognosis for improvement? (We will deal with insurance coverage for this and other costs in following chapters.)*

When Mom's deterioration began, we needed to find out what prognosis, if any, there was for improvement. It never occurred to us prior to a conversation we had with her occupational therapist that she could, in fact, increase her mobility and help herself to do more things for herself. We mistakenly assumed that once the aging process took over she could not reclaim those skills. Her goals were limited, but had she not been in a facility that offered her this help, she would not have improved at all.

For our family, the preservation of Mom's personal dignity was a vital issue. We believe that rehabilitation is a critical element in the maintenance of that dignity. The more an individual can do for himself or herself, the more he or she feels self-confident and independent. Independence feeds the dignity we all associate with being able to care for ourselves.

Medical-related Questions to Ask the Facility

1. Are residents "mainstreamed" or are they segregated by level of care? What is the facility's philosophy of care?

We have borrowed a term from the educational system here. At the facility where Mom lived the longest, all residents ate together. People who had trouble feeding themselves ate alongside those who could better care for themselves. This encourages those with problems as they try to increase their abilities. At another facility we noticed segregated seating which seemed to worsen the problem. There are, as always, two schools of thought on this and you need to decide what is best for your loved one.

This question may give you an idea of some of the care options available. By asking it, you will also learn whether your loved one will be physically moved to another location should the care needed increase dramatically.

> 2. *Do doctors regularly visit the facility? Do dentists? Ophthalmologists? Podiatrists? If not, who provides transportation to appointments? The family? The care center?*

When Mom was in a facility not visited by her doctor, we picked her up and took her to appointments. Because Robin is self-employed and Lonnie's hours are flexible, this posed no significant problems. It can become a major problem, though, for people who have several schedules — work, children, church, etc. — to juggle.

Remember to check with the facility to see what kind of transportation is available. Does the facility have its own transportation? Are there additional charges for this service? Will Medicare or private insurance cover these costs?

> 3. *If these medical professionals do visit the facility regularly how does one make an appointment? Stay informed of the visits? Is any advance notice given? Does the medical professional retain an active role in the care given your family member? Do you?*

Some facilities have Nurse Practitioners who visit their residents regularly. The two women who saw and worked with Mom were godsends to us. In part, because their position was created with this in mind, they were more accessible than the physicians and were also able to help with medication and therapy decisions.

> 4. *Are medications ordered and delivered directly to the care center? How does a family know when medications have changed?*

Because her insurance was accepted by only one pharmacy in our area, we picked up Mom's prescriptions and delivered them to the care center. In that way, we stayed informed of changes and needs for her. If we were asked to get a prescription and we had no idea what it did, took care of or was intended to take care of, we called the doctor, the nurse at the care facility or the nurse practitioner and found out. Again, pharmacists are also a good resource for this.

> 5. *What is the care center policy on patient's rights? Can residents refuse medication? If so, how does the staff respond?*

This was one of the hardest issues we had to deal with. Just as our friends and other family members wanted us to force Mom to accept in-home care, we wanted the nurses and aides at the care center to make Mom take her pills, go to the activities, like the place — in short, be a "good patient." All of that now sounds pompous and condescending. If our love and respect for her was *our* compass, how could we expect or demand anything else from her caregivers? We finally had to remind ourselves of our belief system and follow through with that. This wasn't easy, but it acknowledged Mom's right as a person to make some choices for herself. One shouldn't accept less. Would you?

> 6. *What is the care center policy on emergency measures? Can the resident or family determine what measures, if any, would be taken? If so, how?*

When we checked Mom in to the care center, Robin was asked to determine the level of emergency measures which would be taken if his mother was in a life threatening situation. This must be asked upon admission. The care center has no choice.

Be prepared for this. The best preparation is a Living Will which outlines and defines the patient's preferences. Mom refused to sign any such document, believing, despite numerous explanations, that it somehow affected her finances. In one way we were lucky because Mom had spoken with Robin and his brother about her wishes not to have any heroic measures taken. We were also fortunate in that she had also talked about this with her doctor.

Whatever your specific situation, it doesn't change how difficult it is to sign a document that says you don't want your loved one resuscitated. The information that finally made it easier for Robin was the knowledge that once resuscitative measures had begun, the care center was obligated to transport their resident to a hospital which was, in turn, obligated to continue any procedures already initiated. In practice, this meant that the family would have to decide to request that all artificial life supports be removed after the process had begun rather than never initiate heroic measures at all. It may not seem like much of a choice, but for us it represented a monumental difference.

We were also made aware that limited care does not equal suffering. Measures to ensure a patient's comfort can be taken without resorting to the use of other life support systems. Comfort is always of major importance.

We just mentioned a "Living Will." Check Chapter Seven and the glossary at the end of the handbook for the definitions of this and other documents. You will need to know what you are talking about. Not only do medical professionals have their own language, legal professionals do, too. The more you know, the better off you will be.

7. How does the staff communicate with each other regarding medical treatment?

It doesn't do much good to have asked your doctor and the care center all of these questions if you are not provided with a format and opportunities to maintain communications with the professionals caring for your loved one. At each of the care centers Mom lived in, the staff held regularly scheduled care conferences with nursing, social services, activities, occupational therapy and dietary staff present to discuss her status and/or progress. Make sure the care conferences are scheduled when you can attend, that you receive adequate notification, and that you have enough time to understand all the information you are being given.

It is not always easy to demand these things but you must. If your loved one is ill enough to be placed in a care center, he/she needs an advocate. In all likelihood, your loved one is unable to speak up on his/her behalf. He/she needs reinforcement and confirmation and someone who can and will articulate their special needs. The staff understands, and while they may be understaffed and overworked, they do want to help you and your family member to the best of their abilities. Join together to find a way that works for both of you.

Remember, you know your loved one better than anyone at the facility, and you can help the caregivers as much as they can help you.

And now what do we do?

- Be assertive. Get the answers you need.

- Start with your physician. Find out everything you can about the medical needs of you or your loved one.

- Make sure the care centers you are considering have a physical plant which will meet the medical needs of you or your loved one. Ask about treatment programs as well as the actual living spaces available for residents.

- Talk to your loved one about a "Living Will" or make sure you are fully aware of his or her wishes before the admission process begins. You will be asked for this decision at that time and you will be required to respond.

- Make sure you know the procedures for monitoring medical care of your family member. Ask about everything from medications to care conferences.

The Facility & The Resident Services

Now you have spoken with medical professionals and you have some idea of the care needs of you or your loved one. This will help focus your search for a facility. The following questions were created to help you understand if your family member will have his/her medical needs met at a given care center, if he/she will be comfortable there — both physically and socially — and if the policies and procedures established by the facility will fit the needs of you and your family.

1. What is the date of the most recent visitation by the Health Department and what were the results?

Most importantly, *every* facility must pass an annual examination by the Health Department, and the results of this exhaustive study must be posted at the facility. When you visit the facility, check the posted results and compare them with the information you received over the phone.

2. How large is the facility? How many people live there?

There are several reasons to ask these questions. The first is for you to get an idea of whether you are dealing with a large or small business. Although we will deal with staff and personnel issues in later chapters, you also need to know how many staff people actually care for the residents. Is this facility too large for your privacy-loving father? Are there too many people here for your introverted mother to feel comfortable?

3. *Are there public areas other than a large communal dining room that might provide for options in social interaction? Can residents leave their rooms but still find a quiet place to read or chat or knit or draw or simply rest? Is there an area outside — a park, a garden, a patio — available in good weather?*

4. *What kind of living arrangements are available? Private/single rooms? Double rooms? Rooms with a private bath? A shared bath? Independent living? Assisted living? Round-the-clock nursing care?*

5. *If bathrooms and washrooms are shared, are they shared with residents of the same gender? Are there full bathrooms, half baths?*

These are CRITICAL questions. We knew that Robin's mother was a *very* private person and our first choice was a single room with a private bath. Because we had limited possibilities available we had to compromise on this issue at the first residence in which she lived. Not only was she sharing a room with a "stranger," she also had to share a bathroom with her roommate and two other people from an adjoining room. It never occurred to us to ask if the other people were men or women. We should have asked. This bathroom was shared by two men and two women and although the staff was wonderful about protecting each person's privacy, it was a huge problem for Robin's mother. She was confused enough, but hearing male voices so close deepened her confusion and scared her at times!

Strange as this may sound, try to remember all the things you had to think about as parents or caregivers for young toddlers. Some of those same concerns should be exhibited here. What are your loved one's bathroom habits? Do they like to spend an unlimited amount of time readying themselves for the day? If so, maybe you should consider a private bathroom. This often costs more but if it is important to your loved one it needs to be important to you.

You may have to compromise on one — or several — issues initially as we did, but try to keep all the needs in mind. At the next facility, Mom shared a bathroom with one woman and we put her on a waiting list for a room with a private bath. Eventually she got a private room with a private bath. We were relieved and so was she.

Private rooms may be the preference of your loved one but you also need to talk about whether that is the best living situation for him or her — or you. Private rooms usually cost more and some medical assistance or insurance programs will not cover that extra cost. Perhaps your loved one needs to be motivated to socialize. A roommate can do that. Perhaps they need to have stimulus to engage themselves in the normal activities of a day. A roommate can help an overworked staff do that for another resident simply by being an active person in the same room. Think about all the ramifications. If the facility itself has options, you can start with one type of room and move to another should that prove to be a better living arrangement. If the facility has only one option make sure it's the best option for your family.

6. Are the general showers and baths out of the normal traffic pattern, offering privacy to the residents? What is the bathing schedule?

This is more a privacy question than a hygiene question. You should learn all you can about your loved one's schedule. Here's another example of experience being the best teacher. Robin's mother responded extremely well to having her hair done. She seemed to feel better and wanted to do more on days when she felt she looked better. Feeling smart and efficient, we scheduled her for a weekly appointment at the resident beauty shop — on the day before her weekly shower. Obviously, she resisted bathing because she didn't want to ruin her hair. It only took a week for us to see what we had done, but this is just one reason for the need to understand schedules and what they mean to your plans.

The residence Mom lived in had two bathing facilities, both of which many visitors had to pass to get to residents' rooms. The staff did their best to protect privacy but being there during bathing time can be very awkward for easily embarrassed family members. Again, be aware of this so you don't show up for a visit while your father is having his weekly shower.

> *7. What comes with a room? Can a resident bring furniture from home? Pictures? Are televisions encouraged? Are cable hook-ups available? Is there a lockable drawer in the room where private items can be stored?*

Everyone we talked with at the facility, including residents, family members or staff people encouraged us to make Mom's room as much her home as possible. We agreed. Before her eyesight deteriorated, it meant something to her, too. Our family brought a bulletin board with pictures of relatives, wall hangings, a lamp, a chair and a couple of plants.

Remember to label everything with your family member's name and/or your name and address. Many care centers will also require you to complete an inventory of the items you bring.

The facility will ask you to remove all articles of value, but we brought a purse and some personal things from home. It made Mom feel more in charge of herself, in control of her life, even though the purse contained only a few dollars. Dignity, self-determination and familiarity are important elements of caring for a loved one in a resident facility.

The family gave Mom a small TV for Mother's Day one year. It was a better present than we had imagined. Mom had always enjoyed a few programs, but it was great to watch Chicago Cubs games with her when we visited (hence the need for cable since we live in Minnesota) or remind the nurses to turn on *The Lawrence Welk Show* on Thursday nights. It also gave us something to focus on or talk about if Mom was having a bad day or feeling blue or wanted us to be there but didn't want to talk. Just the mere presence of a loved one or friend was welcomed. Conversation or subject matter was far less important.

If your loved one will have a roommate, you also need to ask about that person's habits or preferences. Does the potential roommate watch TV constantly? Does your loved one hardly ever turn it on? Does the roommate enjoy reading at all hours of the day or night? Does your loved one demand complete darkness in order to sleep? Flexibility is not a common trait in the aging and you need to recognize this when you are examining potential living situations. Even if your choices are limited, do the best you can to find an environment that is as comfortable as possible.

8. *Do residents have private telephones? Do they have access to public phones? Does the staff assist them in making calls?*

Our care center offered residents the option of having a private phone in their rooms. We opted not to do that as we lived in the same town and Mom had access to a phone next door to her room. When her eyesight began to prevent her from dialing on her own, the staff helped her.

It is important that your family members be given the opportunity to communicate with anyone they might choose, but it is also important to consider the effects of their illness. Mom's dementia caused her great confusion. Had she had unlimited or unmonitored access to a phone she might have called the police, the fire department or others — or us — at all hours of the day or night with very confusing accounts of her life and concerns of the moment. We needed to monitor telephone use in order to make sure she got the responses that would help her the most. That is, she needed to talk with someone who knew she was ill. We were that someone and we encouraged the nursing staff to have her call us when she needed to. It seemed to be the right choice for her — and for us.

9. *Is there a laundry? How often are clothes picked up for laundering? How are they returned? Do all articles need to be labeled? Are pick-ups noted with receipts? Is there an additional fee for this service?*

Every care center we contacted needed to have clothes labeled appropriately. Some centers will label clothing for you, but remember that the staff is often overworked and the labeling may therefore not get done in a timely fashion. Everything new that you bring, or that your loved one receives as a gift, should be labeled immediately. It still may get lost, but with a label you at least have a chance to keep track of it.

Laundries in care centers are institutional laundries. If you or your loved one have delicate articles of clothing, wash them yourself.

This is an example of realism in expectations when you deal with a care facility. Don't expect people who do dozens of loads of laundry every day to care about the lace petticoat your mom received from Aunt Freda last Christmas.

10. *How often are the rooms cleaned? Does this include dusting, vacuuming, mopping? Does this include hallways, bathrooms and general visiting areas?*

Every facility must meet a set of state and federal regulations regarding the cleanliness of the entire physical plant and its effect on the residents. We tried to keep that in mind but we also complained when the floor under the bed went unswept for days. It wasn't a health hazard but it bothered Mom and it bothered us. We wanted it fixed and it was. This is, after all, where you or your loved one are living...not just existing. Living.

11. *How secure is the facility? Is there security staff twenty-four hours a day? Can residents feel safe walking the grounds?*

Another central issue. We felt that we should be able to visit at any time we cared to or were needed but we were also willing to meet all the regulations for those visits. A comprehensive security plan is essential for the safekeeping of the residents, the staff and the mental well being of the families. Again, this is a place people are *living*, so we did not want bars on the windows. But we wanted to know that Mom could be inside or outside when she wanted to be, and that she would be safe being there.

12. *How are meals served? Family style? Are seats assigned? Are there selections from a menu? Are snacks brought to individual rooms? Do aides assist in feeding certain residents? Are seconds provided?*

13. *Can families dine with their loved ones? How much notice is required? Are private dining rooms available? Are there additional fees or meal charges? Can they be paid in the dining area? If not, where?*

Meals are often the biggest social event of the day for many residents. The dining facility at Mom's care center was a lovely room with lots of windows and beautiful wallpaper. Places were assigned and the routine was one Mom seemed not only to accept but appreciate.

Families were encouraged to join their residents for meals and 24 hours' notice was encouraged but not required. Private facilities were available for families dining together but we could also join Mom in the main dining area. Special events throughout the calendar year included families and ranged from a Holiday Dinner in December to a Family Reunion Picnic in August.

Once the staff knew that Mom loved ice cream, they tried to make sure she got a special treat in the evenings or for dessert. She was given a snack in the afternoon and we were told to help ourselves to coffee while visiting. We didn't understand how important this relative "freedom" with food was until we realized it was all part of the same life control issues we have already talked about. In her mind, if Mom couldn't even pick what she would or would not eat, then why eat at all? Giving her some options from which she could choose really cost the facility nothing and made her feel much less vulnerable to a group of people "running" her life. Residents could also store a limited number of items in a refrigerator in a secure area. Most common among the items stored there were special flavors of ice cream, some alcoholic beverages, jello and puddings.

14. *Is there a beauty/barber shop?*

15. *What costs are involved with available amenities? Do residents have private "bank" accounts from which they can draw to cover the costs for these services? How are these accounts set up? Are regular reports issued on the balance in these accounts?*

16. *Is there a store from which residents can purchase toiletries, magazines, etc.?*

Amenities such as a beauty/barber shop or a "store" from which toiletries, snacks or cards can be purchased should not be confused with crucial care issues. We include them here because they add to the quality of life a resident experiences at *any* facility. Excursions for a haircut can be a great activity, but knowing they don't need you to take them to get a haircut also empowers your family member to control what he or she can still control.

Each of the two facilities Mom lived in had a personal account system so we could deposit money against which Mom could draw to cover the things she chose to do, whether that was a haircut or a field trip which included lunch. We believe these accounts are very helpful for everyone involved. Your aging loved one doesn't need to try to keep track of a lot of money, the facility doesn't need to worry about the theft of money from residents' rooms, and you can make sure there is always enough for your loved one to do what he or she wants to do without having to ask anyone else. This eliminates the possibility of an embarrassing situation — for your loved one and for you — of being asked for financial assistance to do something as mundane as get a haircut.

17. Is there a resident council to provide feedback to the administration?

Resident councils are another avenue through which your loved one can communicate his or her needs. Their existence tells you that the people who are running this facility want to know if their customers are happy. You might want to ask to read some of the back issues of minutes to determine the nature or character of the council. You can also ask if family members are allowed to attend with their resident. It can be a real treat for both of you to see Mom or Dad "in action" again.

You might want to find out how often the council meets, how many residents are on the council, how they are selected and what staff member meets with them. The answers to these questions will tell you how seriously the concerns of the residents are taken. If the decision-makers on the administrative staff meet with this group, they are serious in monitoring their care in any way they can. That kind of concern can speak volumes about the level of care they deliver.

Finally, don't expect every nurse in the facility to know when your father had his last haircut. Know which staff people care for your loved one and check with them. In our experience, staff people try to meet your needs, but remember who and what you are dealing with. Be realistic in your expectations of the staff, of your loved one and of yourself.

> ### And now what do we do?
>
> - Check the evaluation of the inspection required of every facility by the Health Department. It must be posted in the care center.
>
> - Understand the social and personal needs of your loved one. Know their issues and try to respond to them.
>
> - Make sure the care centers you are considering have a physical plant which will meet the social and personal needs of you or your loved one.
>
> - Understand the schedule at the care center and assist the staff by planning your visits or special events accordingly.
>
> - Respect your loved one's dignity by acknowledging their need to make as many decisions for himself or herself as he/she is capable.
>
> - Understand that emotional and physical comfort must always be a concern in your care or the care of a loved one.

The Personnel 4

By this time, you have a good awareness of the special needs of you or your loved one and the physical plant that will be necessary to meet those needs. Now we come to the often daunting task of evaluating the people who will be your primary caregivers.

Don't shy away from this. It is crucial that you be able to trust the people who will serve as caregivers for you or your family member. You must judge the staff on their background and training but you must also feel comfortable asking them questions, talking to them about problems and relying on their judgment where care is concerned.

There are stumbling blocks to avoid.

First, don't under-analyze the situation or continually defer to the staff members that you are interviewing out of a mistaken notion that you are "just a lay person" and they are nursing professionals who know how to help you solve a serious problem. In other words, don't let gratitude cloud your evaluation.

Second, don't over-analyze their academic or professional training. This is an integral element in the evaluation of the staff as a whole, but you can better judge their qualities as caregivers by watching them in action with the residents under their care.

Third, trust your own reactions. Your ability to communicate effectively and function as part of a *team* of caregivers will impact the quality of life your loved one experiences more than any other single factor.

When we first moved Mom into the care center, we were overwhelmed with forms to sign and questionnaires to answer. Each of these documents came from a different member of the staff. Although everyone was congenial, we were exhausted when we finally felt she was settled enough for us to go home. Within a week or so, we were having a tough time finding answers to Mom's and to our questions. Every time we asked someone something, we were referred to somebody else.

Many small problems that we had left unattended through initial ignorance or gratitude had now become major issues in our minds. A frustrated nurse manager who gave a curt response to a question was the last straw. We were paying a lot of money every month and we expected people to respond to our needs. To the credit of the care center staff, we received a call from the social worker that afternoon. She set up a meeting between us and the nursing team caring for Mom. With candor and kindness, we worked through our communication problems then and there. Regardless of how much money you or the government pays, candor, kindness, communication and mutual respect get better results.

A staff committed to responding to a family's needs is one in which you can place trust. We weathered this storm and came out of it with some real understanding of what it is like to walk in another person's shoes. Concerns need to be addressed immediately and in a respectful manner. This is the basis of good communication and a necessity to develop between you and your loved one's primary caregivers.

Let's start with some of the basics…

1. *How large is the staff? How many of these people have administrative responsibilities? How many are direct caregivers?*

2. *Of the direct caregivers, how many are nurses? Nurses' aides? Nurse practitioners?*

3. What is the nursing staff/resident ratio?

Compare the size of the staff to the number of residents. To get a more accurate picture of the actual workload of people who care for residents, compare the number of staff with direct care responsibilities to the total number of residents. Is there a staff person for every five or six residents? Every 10 or 12? Every 20 or 30?

If this ratio seems too high, you need to think about the needs of you or your loved one. Does he or she require constant monitoring? Are they able to dress themselves? Can they get around by themselves within a confined environment? The more direct care they need, the more concerned you should be about the ratio.

A word of caution. The ratio will always seem too high because no care facility has a one-to-one ratio of staff to residents. Try to understand the way the staff works. Mom's care center was equipped with call lights in each of the residents' rooms and in the public washrooms. Residents were asked to use the call light when they needed any kind of assistance. When a person needs help getting out of bed or to go the restroom, a minute can seem like an eternity. In our experience, it *felt* like the aides took forever to arrive, but it actually happened in a matter of only a few moments. Be realistic. While we felt she was sometimes ignored, we believe her needs were ministered to in a timely manner.

4. How is the nursing staff organized? To whom should questions be directed?

5. *How is the administrative staff organized? To whom should questions be directed?*

In most organizations and, therefore, in most care facilities, there is a reporting structure which assigns responsibilities and authority in some sort of rank order. Find out what the procedures are and follow them.

In some facilities we contacted, there is a Director of Nursing who oversees the activities of the entire nursing staff. Nurse managers are assigned to a set number of nurses and they in turn are given trained assistants to aid them in their efforts. Occupational and physical therapy programs fall outside the responsibilities of these people but the nurse manager keeps track of all special needs for the patients assigned to their "team."

Some facilities want you to call the nurse manager with any questions or concerns. Others ask you to deal with their social workers. As long as there are procedures in place, try to relate them to your expectations and then follow them. If you don't get the answers you need, proceed "up the ladder" until you do. Remember, you have a right – and a responsibility – to understand what's going on at all levels of your own or a loved one's care.

Although it may seem much more obvious when you get to the administrative staff, you should still ask about appropriate procedures. It may seem logical to call the business office with questions about a bill but is that what you should do? When is it advisable to contact the chief administrator? Is he or she normally available to families? The more you know about how the facility operates the better it will operate for you and your loved one.

6. *Is there a social worker? What are the responsibilities assigned to that position?*

In all of the care centers we visited, it was the responsibility of the social worker to meet with the family and talk about the facility, answer questions and, in general, facilitate the admissions process. Social workers also meet regularly with the residents to assess their individual situations. They participate in care conferences and help the resident and the family adjust to any changes in the care or the health of their loved one.

Social workers are a veritable wealth of non-medical information but, as with many of the staff people at these facilities, their case load is often unmanageable. Be assertive and clear about your needs. Do you want to know more about financial assistance? Medicaid? Medicare? Do you need to know more about Living Wills? All of the above? The social worker can and will help you.

If you are looking to the facility's social worker to provide you or your family with some intensive counseling, make sure they are willing and trained to do so. If not, ask for referrals to other professionals who can meet your needs.

Mom's care center has a somewhat informal Family Council. The mission of such a group is to participate actively in the lives of their loved ones and the care center. It also functions as a place where families can go for help and support as they ride the emotional rollercoaster this process often becomes. Support groups also exist outside the confines of those associated with a specific institution. The social worker can help you find the right group for your needs.

> 7. *Is there an activities staff? What are its responsibilities?*

Care facilities that have an activities staff have made a commitment to the social aspect of their residents' lives which must be addressed outside their medical needs. A facility interested in the total resident will have regularly scheduled programs such as church services, entertainment, card games and exercise classes. We will explore some of the specifics in the next chapter.

While Mom wasn't much of a "joiner," she did enjoy activities once she got to them. The staff at her facility went out of their way to come to the residents and help them get to the location of the next event. This really makes a difference to people who have difficulty getting around. It also allows those who are intimidated by meeting new people to enter the room with someone everyone knows. Staff people can then make initial introductions and get people off on the right foot.

> 8. *What is the level of experience and training for staff members having direct contact with the residents? Is there a high priority placed on training and re-training in "people skills," i.e. communications, as well as medical care? Are there provisions for in-service training? Who provides the bulk of the training? the center itself? other professional training centers?*

Training is a critical element in the effectiveness of staff. Not only should the care facility's personnel be well-versed in medical procedures, they must also be able to identify behavior characteristics which directly

• • •

affect the well-being of the resident and the staff's ability to care for that resident.

For example, some residents of a facility may suffer from dementia. Dementia is a physical disorder which affects the ability of the brain to function "normally." People who suffer from this disease are often disoriented and have trouble with short term memory but it affects different individuals in different ways. Staff people who care for dementia patients must understand not only the disease but how it affects the particular patient with whom they are dealing. A staff person who knows when to confront, when to walk away or when to simply listen can be a valuable and integral aspect of the patient's sense of well-being and security. The aide — or housekeeper or laundry person or dietitian or maintenance person — who understands this is a treasure.

Care facilities which make a commitment to training and re-training every level of staff — from administration to medical to food service to maintenance to clerical — have made a commitment to the residents and their families. They understand that they have been entrusted with the life of a special human being. They keep their staff people up to speed to meet the changing physical needs of their residents as well as to meet their social and emotional needs.

Remember, it is the aides or assistants who will answer the call for help your loved one makes at 3 a.m. You need to feel confident that the person who is there to help knows what they are doing and with whom they are dealing.

Staff training scheduled on a regular basis also gives the staff the message that they are trusted employees who are worthy of further education. Valued employees are empowered to perform their tasks to the very best of their abilities. You may not understand all the intricacies of specific training programs, but you will understand if the facility has made a commitment to staff and residents by providing frequent and relevant training.

When these programs are at their best, the dedication extends to all levels of the staff. Our local care facility recently initiated a weekend Customer Service Representative. The top twelve managers at the facility commit one weekend a quarter – for no additional compensation – to working at the care center. They make "rounds," visiting with the residents and having lunch in one of the dining areas. They make sure the mail gets delivered on Saturday and they help with church services. They are also there to give tours to interested families or prospective residents as well as to field any phone calls or non-medical questions which may come up over the course of the two days.

This program has had several positive effects: the residents feel important because the administrators care about talking with them, the nursing staff feels valued by the administration (their work shouldn't be interrupted by tours or other non-emergency needs) and the families and prospective residents get their questions answered in a timely, efficient and accurate manner.

Effective communications start at a rudimentary level and build on these basics. Mom suffered from dementia and failing eyesight. The medical staff at her care center did not wear uniforms but did wear badges which proved to be unreadable for Mom. Since she couldn't recognize people as they entered her room, she had counted on white uniforms to tell her when nurses approached. Unfamiliar with Mom's needs, the staff often did not introduce themselves when they came with medications, etc. When we discovered how uncomfortable this made Mom, we met with the staff and requested they make a simple introductory remark when they came into Mom's room. This seemed like a small thing but it eased her mind and alleviated her unfounded fears.

> *9. What is the staff turnover? What is the average tenure for nursing staff, support staff and administrative positions?*

You will want to know if people like working there. As with any business there are positions which may be less personally fulfilling and, therefore, have a higher turnover rate. But, in general, do they stick around for more than a few months? Is there an employee recognition program?

This is yet another instance when you will need to go on instinct rather than facts. It isn't necessarily good or bad to have many people on staff who have been there for many years. It does say something negative about an organization which cannot retain the majority of their employees for significant periods of time. If something doesn't seem right, ask about it. Was there a mass exodus because a beloved director left? Or because the director was fired as were the staff he or she hired?

> *10. Are employees screened through drug testing? for criminal records, etc.?*

Everyone has heard a horror story about the abuse of residents at a care facility. These stories are the exception, not the rule. But however few and far between, even one case of abuse is one too many. As much as they are legally able, facilities should make sure the people they hire are people who can be trusted with lives. State and federal statutes will govern the nature of this screening, but find out how much can be done and, more importantly, how much is being done.

And now what do we do?

- Become part of the team.
- Avoid the stumbling blocks of too much or too little evaluation. Be realistic.
- Find out the ratio of aides and nursing staff to residents.
- Make sure there is a variety of staff positions to deal with the many needs of residents and their families.
- Check on the training and background of the staff as well as the training offered to them on a regular basis.
- Make sure some attention is given to personal communications skills as well as to proficiency in medical procedures.
- Understand the organization of duties and responsibilities and find out where you should go for any problem or question you may have.
- The more you know about how a facility operates, the better it will operate for you and your loved one.

Social Activities

At the core of any search for the right care facility is a concern for the quality and dignity of life of the individual who will be residing there. Whether you are investigating possibilities for yourself or a loved one, you must always remember that a person will be *living* in this place with these people. The more aware you are of personal preferences, medical needs and personal habits, the better your choice will be.

> 1. *What activities or range of activities are regularly planned for the residents?*

The variety of care needed for residents at any care center will cover a broad spectrum. Residents may need short-term recuperation and physical rehabilitation from surgery or they may require full time nursing care for the remainder of their lives. The activities planned should cover as wide a range of needs as the residents' care demands.

The scheduled activities don't need to be elaborate to be effective. At the care facilities we have visited, weekly bridge games are on the same schedule as performances by the local youth choir. There are Bible studies and church services – both ecumenical and denominational. There are speakers who talk about interesting trips they have taken and arts and crafts sessions where residents can create items for themselves or for family gifts. The point is variety. No one resident will probably attend everything but there should be something on the schedule your loved one will find interesting.

Activities get people out of their rooms and, for a few moments, take a person's mind off their troubles and ailments. Many care facilities also schedule "off-campus" shopping trips or excursions to a play, a movie or a museum. Even residents who have some ambulatory problems can enjoy these programs if they are prepared for the trip and have some dedicated assistance. These trips may cause some trauma for residents who are easily confused or upset when their environment changes. Before you encourage your loved one to participate in any activity, know his or her limitations and accept them. Activities won't do anyone any good if they are entered into defensively or reluctantly.

Some care centers also encourage visits by children from nearby day-care facilities. The kids and their new grandparent-like friends can create art work together, have ice cream together or simply enjoy each other's company. There are also programs that schedule visits of domesticated animals for the facility. Pets and children are totally accepting of the residents and offer them unconditional enjoyment as well.

2. Who manages the activities? How often do they occur?

In the last chapter, we talked briefly about professional activities staff people who manage the more social aspects of living in a care center. If the facilities you are considering do not employ full or part-time activities staff, find out how they manage these programs if they exist at all. Volunteer-driven activity programs can be very well run but they are also subject to the availability of the volunteers managing them. Staff-run schedules tend to be much more regular and the residents respond very well to this consistency.

There should also be some facility-supported programming which encourages the participation of other family members. Family dinners at holidays or special projects can be a heartwarming experience for everyone involved. An annual family picnic is just one example of the type of program which can turn into a family tradition. This will never completely replace more traditional family events but it can go a long way toward helping maintain family ties through the separation which occurs when a loved one enters a care center.

> *3. Are residents allowed to pursue hobbies (cooking, writing, sewing, etc.)? Are they drawn into the operation of the facility by being asked to help with mailings or to act as "host or hostess for the day?"*

This may seem like a small thing, but the ability to pursue lifelong pleasures can make a significant contribution to the residents' sense of well-being. Be prepared to volunteer your time and energies to help with this pursuit. The care center may provide all the equipment necessary, but there are often no staff people able to devote a lot of time to activities which do not interest the majority of the residents.

Some care facilities have craft sales run by the residents. Any money earned is contributed to a cause or program determined by the participants. No matter what the amount, an activity of this type is an ego-booster and very beneficial to the organization which receives the proceeds.

When residents are asked to help with bulk mailings, answer phones or perform other clerical support functions for the care center, they respond very positively. Some care centers ask residents to serve as host or hostess to that day's visitors. Monitored by the social services staff, these volunteers often provide a wonderful first impression to anyone entering the center for the first time.

Activities that provide a sense of ownership in their surroundings help give aging citizens a sense of their ability to contribute to their "home." Every resident experiences the vulnerability which failing health and mental capabilities inflict. Anything that can be done to alleviate feelings of uselessness should be given the highest priority.

4. Are there opportunities for group or individual worship services? Is there regular visitation by denominational clergy or volunteers?

We have mentioned church services frequently when talking about activities. The opportunity to attend some form of organized service is extremely important to many aging residents. If you or your loved one have selected a facility that is supported by a denomination or religious tradition other than yours or his/her own, you will want to make sure other worship options are available. Sometimes local churches or synagogues regularly schedule visits by the pastor, rabbi or a lay volunteer. For some residents, this one-on-one contact may be preferable to a more formal service.

Although we were unaware of the program, our church enlisted volunteers who identified church members (or members of their families) who were residents of our three local care facilities and visited with them on a regular basis. Mom would often tell us the "church lady" had visited. Since we had never met such a volunteer, we at first assumed Mom might have imagined the visit, or that the center's chaplain had been there. When we began finding our church's newsletters in Mom's room, we did a little checking and found out who was visiting and when. Our visits had just never overlapped.

This is a perfect example of the many thoughtful, compassionate acts which affect the life of a family member in a care center. You may never meet the people who are showing kindness to your loved one. Eventually, we were able to thank the "church lady" personally, but there are many other gifts we were never able to acknowledge. Every act, every visit was truly helpful and greatly appreciated.

5. *Are pets allowed or encouraged?*

When care centers offer a variety of living options, small, non-threatening and socially adjusted pets are often encouraged. In situations where you or your loved one require more than cursory medical supervision, pets may be discouraged or forbidden. Some centers have aviaries or aquariums which are often cared for and "stocked" by the residents. If having a pet is a critical issue for you or your loved one, you will need to explore all of your options. Contact with animals is often therapeutic and usually well accepted.

The Nurse Manager at Mom's care center brought her small cocker spaniel to work every day. A dog lover, Mom got a kick out of the daily visits she and the other residents were paid.

6. *Are there opportunities for young children to interact with the residents?*

Family visitation is rarely restricted unless health concerns dictate. If you have young children you want to bring with you on your visits to a loved one, make sure you know everyone's schedule. Limit your visit to the time your child is content. Noisy running through the halls or other normal, child-like behavior can be disruptive to other residents or, in fact, to your own family member. Kids need to be kids. It is their energy and joy of living that makes them wonderful visitors in care centers. If you are careful about the time you select to visit, it can be an uplifting experience for everyone.

Babies are particularly welcome at many centers. For many residents, these tiny people take them away from their aches and pains. It is soothing and heartwarming to watch them cradle a child. Here they find a human being more vulnerable than they for whom they can be a protector. This also happens with small pets. No wonder these visits can be therapeutic for everyone involved.

As we have stated, some centers cooperate in regularly scheduled visitation programs with local daycare centers. Youth service organizations should also be encouraged to visit and participate in activities of their own or the center's choosing.

7. Are activities scheduled for all times of the day, including in the evening after dinner?

Every adult body ages differently. Individuals who longed for retirement so they could sleep until noon find themselves awake at 6 a.m. People who went to bed by ten o'clock every night find themselves awake and alert at 1 a.m. Although many care center residents are on a schedule which provides for an early bedtime, some people relish evening activities and interaction with others.

Activities scheduled outside the normal workday are often difficult to staff, but many volunteer organizations can fill this gap by providing evening programs for residents and their families. If you or your loved one is a night owl, make sure you find out what is available after the evening meal. If the center doesn't provide much, perhaps this is the time to schedule family visits. Again, know the center's schedule and your loved one's preferences, and work with both to resolve potential problems before they happen.

> ### And now what do we do?
>
> - Care centers are places people LIVE.
>
> - Find out as much as you can about programs and activities which enhance the quality and dignity of life at the facility.
>
> - People who are given the opportunity to participate in the management or maintenance of their environment are less vulnerable and have a greater sense of well being.
>
> - Know your loved one's preferences and know the programs and policies of the care facility. Work together with your family and the staff to help create a schedule that meets your needs.

Family Services

This chapter has been labeled "Family Services" but it could really be called "Services *for* Families" or "Services *from* Families." Here's why.

In preceding chapters we have spoken briefly about Family and Resident Councils and opportunities for family participation in the life of the resident. We have also mentioned the importance of care conferences and persistent, assertive questioning on the part of you, the resident's advocate. The critical element in every interaction among the family, the resident and the staff is the willingness of each to be a full participant in the process.

Reality dictates that such will not always be the case. Late in our experience of sharing our home with Mom we discovered the local Adult Day Care program. These programs offer marvelous respite for family caregivers and boast a modest cost compared to care center living. They are staffed by nursing professionals and trained assistants. Transportation to and from the program is often readily available and the hours are established to be convenient for people who work at jobs outside their home or for those who have other schedules to maintain (e.g., a child's school play or soccer practice). Mom was unwilling to participate because she refused to be on "anyone else's schedule." We understand now that this was not born out of obstinacy as much as it was out of vulnerability, but her refusal stood. Had we been more assertive in our search for respite alternatives and mentioned this to her before her health began to fail so rapidly, things might have been different.

The point is that you must *actively* seek information. In our work on this project we garnered information on assistance from associations and senior federations and coalitions of which we were completely unaware.

We didn't know about this potential for assistance because the people with whom we came into contact did not tell us, the library and other public resources did not have the information and we were totally unaware of the existence of places like the Office of the Ombudsman on Aging.

We were not kept in the dark because the people we thought would inform us of these kinds of programs were thoughtless or uncaring. Social services people in care centers are grossly overworked as are the nursing staff. Associations are lax in getting their message into public forums where specific information is easily accessible. Family caregivers flounder in the undertow of emotions and immediate needs and find themselves exhausted and frustrated at the end of the day.

All of those factors would fall under the category of good reasons, but this situation is potentially harmful to the unaware families it affects. Check Chapter Ten for more information on associations you might contact and on resources available to you. **No one will do this for you.** If you want to know more about your loved one's options you must be the one to gather that information. There are people out there to help you but, in the end... tag, you're it.

The care centers we saw were all very concerned about the families of their residents. You need to look for the manifestations of that concern. Don't be embarrassed about asking questions regarding programs that will help you and the rest of your family. Just because your loved one is now in a facility, it doesn't meant that you are not part of their care. The more active you are, the better it will be for them.

1. *Who is responsible for maintaining contact with the family?*

This is part of finding out who to talk to about what, and when to do it. Should you contact the social worker with plans for an excursion for your loved one or should you be talking to the nurse manager? If you want to have lunch there, do you call the front office? As simple as these questions sound, the answers will give you peace of mind and eliminate wild goose chases that are energy draining and frustrating.

2. *Is there a Family or Advocacy Council? If so, who participates? Is it active? Is there a newsletter?*

Family Councils can offer you a place to gather information about everything from the administration of the care center to an in-depth look at a disease afflicting your loved one. The best councils are those that seek to offer useful programming on concerns facing families (e.g., legal, support groups for care providers, Medicare and Medicaid regulations, etc.) while providing access to administrators on a regular basis. If the Family Council at a facility is relatively inactive, you can always change that through your own participation.

Our care facility also provided a monthly newsletter to all the residents, but if Mom's was not out in plain sight we often missed seeing it until very late in the month. The newsletter included minutes from the Resident Council meetings, thoughts from the staff, a list of that month's resident birthdays and a calendar of activities. The Family Council, after realizing the newsletter was not mailed to family members, urged the center to mail information to families using the newsletter format and that has been very successful.

Again, you need to know if this project is supported by the staff. Does it function in an ineffective vacuum or do the decision-makers at the facility listen attentively to the concerns expressed by the Family Council? This positive corroboration is critical to the ability of the Council to support the care facility, effect change when needed and advocate for the residents they represent.

> 3. *Are there regular meetings with the nursing staff? Are care conferences scheduled at times when family members can attend? Do families understand what these conferences are intended to cover and accomplish?*

Care conferences are required by law but they are not held solely to dispense information to the family and the resident. It is at these meetings that the overall condition, needs and care of an individual are discussed by everyone who implements and affects that care. At our facility, residents and families were encouraged to attend, but the conferences were not re-scheduled if family members could not participate.

For reasons we have stated before, attendance at mid-morning or mid-afternoon conferences was not a problem for us, but if it is for you be sure you know who to contact to receive a report from the conference. These meetings cover treatments, progress, prognosis, care strategies, and the role everyone — including family members — can play. If you miss the opportunity for interchange with your loved one's caregivers in this forum, find out how you can make your concerns known.

Whenever possible, all three of us attended the conference. Mom would sometimes tire noticeably, but her presence was important to us and to her. When we arrived for one early morning conference, Mom

. . .

was running late. We went down to let everyone know and were informed we only had 15 minutes for the whole meeting as the staff had a big meeting they must attend. We asked why our conference hadn't been rescheduled. We were upset and surprised by the situation and let our feelings be known. The nurse manager recognized we were in need of information and remained at the conference and addressed our concerns patiently and professionally. This problem with bad scheduling never happened to us again.

Had we not been assertive, fifteen minutes of professional jargon would have fulfilled the facility's obligation for the conference. While this situation was unusual, the conferences are only held quarterly and we would have missed an important opportunity to glean significant information about Mom's situation. We looked to the care conferences to provide us with the information our other family members wanted — even demanded — to know.

4. Are there family support groups?

Support groups should not be confused with meetings of the facility's Family Council. Although the Council gatherings often provide emotional support on shared concerns, support groups are focused on the needs of the people who attend. At Mom's care center, there is an Alzheimer's Support Group which meets regularly. The Family Council is also trying to start another group that is envisioned to be much more general in scope.

If a support group is what you seek, don't be hesitant to look beyond the facility. Many communities have groups which meet regularly.

Associations — like the Alzheimer's Association — often sponsor groups of this type as well.

> 5. *Are there opportunities for the family to participate in activities with the residents, such as worship services? Birthday parties? Holiday celebrations? Can families plan excursions outside the facility?*

Every facility we contacted offered families the chance to participate in special events with their loved ones. At Mom's care center, they often plan celebrations with families in mind. To name only a few, there are mother-daughter banquets, holiday parties and birthday celebrations.

Private family gatherings can often be arranged in a private lounge at the care facility. Holidays may pose a problem for the resident and the family. Family members want their loved one at home for the holidays but residents find it disconcerting to be amidst so much activity. Families often find it more meaningful to visit their loved one at the care facility, bringing with them favorite holiday foods and presents, then return home for the remainder of their holiday celebration. As family members, we don't want to believe that would be enough for our mother or grandmother or father or grandfather but it often meets their needs completely.

This brings up a point we must stress. Know whose needs you are meeting when you plan events or schedule things for your loved one. You may miss their constant presence at the holidays but they may be completely incapable of participating at the level you desire. You may want your mother's hair done for her birthday but she may find it a painful experience. Motivations that meet your needs for involvement or for emotional support are not inherently unworthy, but they may set you up for disappointment and you need to be prepared for the response that may come your way. As always, stay in touch with your emotions and needs, and you will be better able to meet the needs of your loved one.

Families can also make their normal visits to their loved one more meaningful by taking their loved one out for a visit. Even a short drive around town or a walk or a wheelchair ride around the grounds can be a welcome change in a resident's routine. It also gives you a focus for the time you spend together.

You may also want to contact the activities staff and find out what type of interaction your loved one seems to enjoy the most. Those activities may not be the ones you would imagine. Don't fall into the trap of making assumptions about someone else's wishes. Even though your dad may have loved singing all his life, he may have opted out of the resident choral group and chosen instead to listen to the local barbershop quartet every time they visit.

> 6. *How are volunteers used? Resident care? Office support staff? Newsletter production? Support group leaders? Are they trained?*

This question is important to you for two reasons. You need to know who is caring for your loved one and you need to know what opportunities there are for you to participate in the broader work of the care center. Volunteer coordinators at many facilities can help you find the right activity. They can also explain the roles the volunteers play at the center.

We found volunteers to be worthwhile additions to the care center community. Not only did they do wonderful things like decorate for the holidays but they also had the time to stop and chat with residents and share a little of their day. They were perceived as "partners in care" by the staff and their roles were considered integral to the successful operation of the facility.

> ## And now what do we do?
>
> - *Actively* seek information.
>
> - Address your needs as well as those of your loved one. Recognize whose needs you are addressing.
>
> - Participate in the life of the facility through Family or Advocacy Councils or as a volunteer.
>
> - Be creative when you plan your visits to the center. Seek the help of the staff to find out schedules for special events or to identify which activities your loved one seems to enjoy the most.

Costs, Funding and Legal Concerns

Every care facility has its own financial policies. Two seemingly identical facilities may approach these matters in two distinctly different ways. Because paperwork requirements and governmental regulations can vary on an almost daily basis, we must remain somewhat general in the terms we use here. Unless you are an attorney or accountant or care center worker specializing in government funding regulations, you will not remember everything. Take notes and ask questions. It's the only way to create the possibility for effective maneuvering through the maze.

1. *What are the costs to a resident? How are these costs determined?*

In our state, the cost of care is determined in large part by the level of care demanded. In turn, the level of care is determined by a thorough, time-consuming evaluation process. The first evaluation is done by a doctor. This is a standard physical, and since many residents come to care centers directly from the hospital, their medical needs are usually clear. The nurses at the care center then do their own evaluation, which is submitted to the state. The state reviews these documents and a care level is established. In our state, "A" is designated as the level for the least amount of care, and "K" is designated as the level where nearly constant, trained nursing care is needed. Mom entered the center at a "G" level.

Each level carries a range of daily fees which can be charged, and every facility in the state must fit their initial charges within this range. (These fees are reviewed and determined by the state Department of Human Services annually. They are based on the facility's previous operating costs.) This helps give one an idea of what the basic costs for this care are going to be statewide. However, you must also ask what is and is not included in that basic fee. In most of the situations we encountered, private rooms were extra, as were private rooms with private baths. In addition, none of the rehabilitation programs were included in the basic fee. Medicare did cover these costs for us but the costs also varied from facility to facility. Make sure you understand what is included and what is not.

> *2. What is the care center's policy on payment? Must a resident reveal all of his or her assets upon admission to the facility? What is the center's billing cycle? What should a family do as assets decline?*

Neither the for-profit nor the non-profit centers in which Mom lived required any formal documentation of her ability to pay. We were asked if there were enough funds to cover at least 90 days of residency without applying for Medical Assistance. Since there were, we then proceeded to the next set of questions. Had she needed Medical Assistance immediately, both centers' social workers were prepared to help us complete all the appropriate paperwork.

Some facilities require much more documentation and much more financial commitment up front. Your loved one may be asked to sign over all of his or her assets prior to admission. In some cases, especially assisted living facilities, your loved one may be asked to purchase outright their own individual living unit in the facility. Costs vary dramatically. We will talk more about asset management later in this chapter.

Also of concern is the actual payment procedure. Are the residents billed and the statements sent to the family? Is a deposit required? If the resident changes facilities, how are the billing changes managed? Who is the facility person responsible for billing and can you contact them to answer your questions? Find out if the credits received from government programs coincide with the billing cycle. In other words, is there a delay in reporting these credits? How does that affect the monthly payment?

Financing long-term care is a costly process. Planning is essential to the effective management of any resources you or your loved one have available. As funds dwindle, it is important for you to know the eligibility requirements of the assistance programs for which you could apply. Ask your county social worker to help you understand the process or ask the social worker at your care center to direct you to the right people. Most importantly, keep the communication channels with your care center open. Let them know of your need for assistance and keep them updated regarding any applications.

> 3. *How is the facility funded? For-profit? Non-profit?*

> 4. *What percentage of funds are received from Medicaid and Medicare? State programs like Medical Assistance? Local or private funds? What is the latest forecast for maintaining these levels?*

These are questions you may not find yourself asking until after your loved one has been admitted to a facility, but they are critical ones nonetheless. Facilities which rely predominantly on state and federally funded programs are subject to the rules of Congress and state legislatures. We did not inquire into a facility which did not receive government funds, but we learned that those which had other financial support were better able to weather the storms of any political climate.

Try to find out what future cost projections are. It may not affect you or your loved one in the next month, but significant cost increases should not be surprises to residents or their families. Costs will always rise but you need to know the general financial condition of the facility you are considering before you make any long term commitments.

You also need to understand the difference between your approach to these fees and that of your loved one. Depression-era residents will have a definite point of view when it comes to financial values. The expense of long term health care can cause high anxiety and be a point of much frustration. Try to help your loved one understand what values they are getting for their dollars. It will help them relax.

Your interest in public plans for changes in Medicare, Medicaid and Social Security will heighten considerably when the reality of cuts in the funding of these programs becomes clear. Even those who pay their own way are affected. Educate yourself in not only the current policies but their effect on you and yours. The same goes for proposed changes. Make sure the Family Council and the staff at any facility you investigate are committed to actively protecting the funds which care for your loved one and his or her peers.

> 5. *Will the care center staff assist the family in obtaining appropriate reimbursement or payments from agencies such as Social Security? Medicare? Medicaid? Medical Assistance? Private insurance?*

The professional nursing staff at Mom's care center took care of all Medicare and Medicaid documentation for Mom. Because her private insurance carried prescription coverage and because that coverage changed in the middle of her stay, we filed all of those claims personally. We also filed two applications for reimbursement from her private insurance but other than that, all of that paperwork was handled by the facility.

This is an often underrated service. If you have not seen a Medicare reporting form, you have missed a life experience. The form is confusing and complicated. No wonder many seniors find themselves with a new career whose primary goal is the interpretation of their Medicare forms. Finding someone who understood what was going on, could explain it in language that was understandable to lay people like us and who would file the actual claim was a blessing. We were so trusting of the staff that we did not request copies of their filings, nor did we ever need to.

At the time of this writing, Medicare will pay for many of the major services in a skilled nursing facility. Those services include a semi-private room, meals, regular nursing services, rehabilitation service, blood transfusions, medical supplies, use of a wheelchair or walker and ex-ray and laboratory services. The requirements surrounding any benefits provided are so complex that errors can and do occur frequently. If you or your loved one are denied benefits, you have the option to appeal decisions. Enlist the support of an advocate like your care facility or the state office of Ombudsman for the Aging.

6. Does your loved one have a will? A Living Will? Does anyone in your family have power of attorney for your loved one?

Both of these questions will be asked of you and your loved one within the first few minutes of your admission interview. You will need to have an answer.

There is a significant amount of difference in these two documents. A person's will usually outlines their specific desires for the distribution of their estate. It will also clarify who will administer that estate and how the distributions should occur. It is a good idea for everyone to have such a document which is accurate and in order legally. Without a will, your loved one's possessions will be distributed according to the laws of the state you live in. Neither they nor their family will have control over this distribution. That lack of control becomes another issue of human dignity which you can help to address.

A Living Will outlines an individual's wishes about being kept alive by medical life support systems in the event of a terminal illness or any other drastic change in their physical health. Facilities are required to provide new residents with written information on Living Wills and other "advance directives." Samples are available through social services. If your loved one does not have a Living Will and if she or he exhibits a lack of ability to make this decision and you are responsible for their well being, you will be asked to make this decision for them.

At the very least, try to have this conversation in the presence of other family members or your loved one's physician, nurse or the care facility's social worker. Intellectually, making this decision is the logical thing to do at this point in your loved one's life. Emotionally, it is as wrenching as though you were signing away their life. We were lucky in that we fully understood Mom's wishes, as did her physician. She refused to sign a Living Will but she did make the needed decision for herself…and, as we discovered, for her family.

Power of attorney is a legal instrument which authorizes someone to act as another's attorney or agent. If the document states that the power will continue to be valid even if the principal (your loved one) becomes incompetent or incapable of making a decision, it is called a durable power of attorney. For the purposes surrounding the placement of a loved one in a care facility, the document you create should be the latter variety. This is a powerful tool and it can help family caregivers tremendously when the family member is unable to make decisions for whatever reasons. The instrument is fairly standard. We received a sample document from the social worker at the care facility.

Even after signing a durable power of attorney, your loved one still has control over his or her life as long as he or she is competent. This is a crucial element to communicate to people who are feeling particularly vulnerable and at everyone else's mercy.

Mom was VERY wary of signing anything that took power away from her or her designated agent. She had made many decisions about the management of her assets prior to this point in her life and she believed she had been very clear about all of her desires. That worked out for our family and it may work in yours. The risk can be very great, however, and as a caregiver you should also be making decisions that are right for your loved one and for you and the rest of your family. If we had asked her to consider this at an earlier, more healthy time, it might have been better received. She also could have been angry. Only you can know what is best for you, your loved one and the other members of your family. What you must understand are the ramifications of those decisions made now; and then, as your loved one's health care needs change, what decisions may be required to fulfill the new demands.

There isn't a time in your life when honesty is more important than this one. You and your siblings, your ailing loved one and other involved family members must find a way to agree about what action is needed and then create a plan to meet those needs. Share your concerns candidly and thoughtfully. The consensus you achieve is worth any time it takes to create it. A united family makes for a supportive family and that can only help your loved one.

> 7. *Have you or your loved one made arrangements to manage financial assets in a manner appropriate to ensure medical care? Personal preferences? Family needs?*

> 8. *What are the current regulations governing this management and how can we find out about them?*

> 9. *How can we plan ahead effectively?*

Individuals and their families who have financial assets of any significance need to make decisions about how they are managed. This is where the waters become cloudy and the sea gets rough. Qualifying for government programs (to which the vast majority of senior citizens believe they are rightfully entitled no matter what their financial status) is directly affected by the assets any individual has. Some individuals try to manage those assets in ways which guarantee inheritances to their children. Some are resigned to using all the funds they have to provide for their care as long as they are able.

Among the variety of financial management tools available to your family are trusts, joint checking or savings accounts or guardianship or conservatorship proceedings. Any of these may meet your needs and could prove useful to you.

A trust is a legal arrangement that gives one person or institution (the trustee) legal title to the assets of another person (the beneficiary) in order for the trustee to manage those assets in a way that is helpful to the beneficiary. The person who creates the trust is called a grantor. A trust can be set up in a will or it can be a living trust, set up during the grantor's lifetime. It is the living trust that gives your family the most flexibility when dealing with managing funds for a person who has become incapacitated. Trusts can be revocable or irrevocable, and are further discussed in Chapter Nine.

Bank accounts held in joint tenancy, where any of the parties designated on the account can make deposits or withdrawals, are also a useful tool. Other accounts can have authorized signers who are not, as with joint accounts, owners of the account. There are also accounts that name one or more people to automatically own the account when the principal dies, thereby eliminating the need for probate. These are sometimes called "in trust for" accounts.

To us, the whole concept of conservatorship seemed far too drastic for our situation. That is an emotional reaction, however, and there are times when families cannot afford the luxury of emotional response alone. If a person becomes incapable of making decisions, handling finances and caring for themselves, a conservatorship may be the best alternative to get his/her life back in order. You must petition to be your loved one's conservator and you can be appointed to this position whether your loved one wants you to be or not. Some families plan for this and establish a conservatorship prior to its need by creating the appropriate legal document. This gives control and power to your loved one and offers them a real voice in their future.

For those of us able to plan ahead, some consideration should be given to long-term care insurance. These policies pay a daily benefit that helps defray care facility expenses. That benefit can be paid for as short a time as one year or until the policyholder dies. This is not a suitable option for people with limited assets who can expect Medicare and Medicaid to cover their costs of long-term care.

Whatever your situation, we suggest you consult an attorney well-versed in this field. Regulations which can affect your loved one's eligibility for Medical Assistance or other programs are complex and may change without your knowledge, but all the ones we encountered were concerned with our family's management of our financial assets.

The best management plan is the plan that starts many years before it is needed. This is a difficult issue to raise with your loved one, but the momentary embarrassment or unease involved with this conversation far outweighs the problems which lack of planning can cause. Regulations change constantly, but doing nothing will ensure that no one's wishes are fulfilled. A professional who is familiar with all the legalities of the system is an invaluable resource. If you don't have an attorney, check with the state ombudsman's office or ask the care facility to suggest some names. It will be money well spent.

You can also get an idea of the current regulations from the social worker at the care facility or county human services offices. A call to the Social Security Administration may also be helpful.

We would like to stress that approaching financial planning with a "beat the system" mentality is a big mistake. As with anything, you need to find the compromise that will best suit your needs and meet the financial responsibilities that accompany quality care.

And now what do we do?

- Take it one step at a time.

- Find out the specifics of what the care center requires. You need to know everything about the financial requirements which will be made of your loved one.

- Plan ahead. Talk with your aging loved one about wills, living wills, financial assets and their wishes for the management of those assets.

- Contact a professional who can help you navigate the waters of fiscal responsibility.

- Know the regulations which govern your financial behavior. If you can't figure out what they are, hire a professional who can.

- Be responsible to your loved one, your family and the care center.

Visiting the Facility

For those of you who aren't hundreds, or even thousands of miles away, the personal visit to a care center can be the most beneficial aspect of all this information gathering. In fact, you may want to visit a facility before you or your loved one even needs to, so the first entry into this world won't be so traumatic. This pre-visit would also offer your loved one a real voice in the decision. Care centers and their staffs are used to such excursions and they welcome your visit and your questions.

Whatever the timing of your visit, the questions and your concerns need to focus on the same core issue — is this the place your loved one should live? The questions which follow, along with those we have already mentioned, should provide you with the best picture available of the facilities you are considering.

1. Are you made welcome or do you feel your visit is an inconvenience?

You should be made to feel welcome when you visit whether that visit is announced or unannounced. However, you also need to remember that you and your concerns come after those of the residents. The staff is there to care for the people who live there. If they can't drop everything immediately, don't take this the wrong way. Try to understand what is going on around you.

You also need to talk with the correct staff person. We found that the social worker was often the staff person everyone met initially. Make sure you are in the "right" office at the center you visit. Ask with whom you should be speaking.

2. Are you spoken down to or deemed reasonably intelligent?

As with any profession, the health care industry has its own vocabulary. Most of us are not well-versed in the language and it can be extremely difficult to understand when spoken "at" you. If the person talking with you is doing this, ask them to stop and talk so that you can understand. In all likelihood, they don't even know they are doing it.

3. Are your concerns listened to or are you given "canned" responses?

Admittedly, most of our questions and most of those that you will ask have been asked before. Still, this does not excuse inattention, condescension or boredom on the part of the staff member with whom you are speaking, and you should not tolerate it. This is one of the most important decisions you will ever make. Although you and your loved one always have the option to change residences, do not approach your decision with an "I can always move" attitude. That would be like agreeing to get married because you know you can always get divorced.

Your concerns are valid and should be taken seriously no matter how much they mirror the concerns of the family who visited right before you. If your specific needs are not addressed, this speaks volumes for your future relationship with the staff.

*4. Are you comfortable with the environment? The furnishings?
The cleanliness of the facility? The cleanliness of the residents?
The staff attitudes toward residents? Toward each other?*

On our tours, we asked to see everything from the room options — single, double, etc. — to the main dining area. We were also shown special areas like the rehabilitation unit and lounges on the individual wings. In neither of the places Mom lived were there problems with cleanliness of the facility, the furnishings or, more importantly, the residents. Nothing and no one showed any signs of neglect — benign or otherwise. This told us that the staff cared not only about appearances but about their residents as individuals and the center as the environment in which they lived. It acknowledged the human dignity of each of the residents and did not go unnoticed by either of us.

The staff communication that impressed us the most was the effort to talk with residents directly. In other words, staff would kneel at the side of residents confined to wheelchairs to make sure they were at eye level. There was no unnecessary raising of voices and no misplaced amusement at the expense of someone having problems navigating a hallway. All levels of staff who had contact with residents seemed to have this attitude. That indicated effective training and a compassionate staff.

You should also be aware of how the staff communicates with each other. Does there seem to be an environment in which an exchange of information is easy and frequent? Does the staff look relaxed? If your guide on the tour of the facility doesn't know an answer is he or she reluctant to ask a colleague?

5. Does the staff seem accessible to residents?

Do the residents seem comfortable in dealing with staff? Are they able to ask questions or chat with staff in an informal way? Are there any casual conversations between staff and residents?

Remember to place these observations in context. If you have arrived during an emergency, you will see none of the informal communication we describe. Staff people will be dealing directly with the emergency or comforting residents so they are not alarmed.

6. *How are the residents addressed? Mr. or Mrs.? By first name? By diminutives such as "dear" or "honey"?*

After Mom had been a resident for a few weeks, a new aide began to work with her. Mom seemed to be irritated by the aide but she couldn't or wouldn't say why. We decided Mom would take care of it if it got really bad, so we let the concern take a back seat to others. One day, Lonnie happened to be visiting when the aide came in to help Mom dress. Not only did she refer to her as "honey," she also completely disregarded Mom's choices of the clothes she wanted to wear that day. Lonnie spoke with the nurse manager immediately. The next time the aide came into the room, she addressed Mom as "Evelyn" and was much more sensitive to human dignity issues like the selection of one's wardrobe. Mom's level of irritability diminished considerably.

While we may not have noticed this on a visit, we realized that more than one of the aides called residents "honey" or "dear." That is fine only if it is fine with the resident or if it is used as a term of affection and not an appellation in place of a person's name. You know what your preferences are and you can tell the difference in the use of these words. Be aware that it is the aides who have the most contact with your loved one. They have a monumental effect on the daily lives of the residents and they need to meet your loved one's needs and standards of behavior. Pay special attention to their interaction with the residents whenever you visit.

7. Are you introduced to staff and/or other residents? Are you given a satisfactory amount of time to get all the information you need?

We met several residents when we visited care centers. Frankly, they were able to answer only simple questions coherently, but they all expressed satisfaction with their living situation and with the staff that cared for them. The willingness of the staff to have people meet and talk with the residents was very telling. The staff members were proud of their work and they were proud of the people they cared for.

The time given to us was also totally dependent upon our needs. While we were aware of the pressing demands on their time, the social workers with whom we spoke never gave us the impression that our time was up. Nursing staff members with whom we spoke were called away to care for patients but they soon returned to complete our conversation. In an emotional moment, this kind of concern for us and, through us, for Mom was much needed and much appreciated.

Again, be realistic. While you may need to be comforted or to ask your questions for hours, you must remember that the concerns of the current residents of any facility come first. If that is not the case, it is cause for you to worry.

If we were to encapsulate all of the questions we have outlined here and in previous chapters, they could be summed up with the question

"Are you and your loved one given quality care and treated with dignity and respect?"

People who enter care facilities are in need of help. Their families are in need of help. Both are often vulnerable and confused. At this time it is crucial to find the health care professionals who will acknowledge these needs and address them. Beyond the fear, the physical pain and the anxiety to do the "right thing" is the understanding that everyone involved is talking about someone's LIFE. This is not an abstraction. It is real and raw and wrenching.

It is tempting to think that in the best of all worlds, this cloak would be taken from our shoulders and those of our family. For most of us, the best of all worlds is the one in which we live — however imperfect. For this world, for this time, we hope this handbook offers you help and solace, and that you or your loved one finds a place in which life can be lived with grace, dignity and love.

And now what do we do?

- If at all possible, visit the care centers you are considering.
- Be observant of everything. Take notes.
- Ask all the questions you have and if you don't understand the answers ask them again until you do.
- Be realistic. Do not expect too much or too little of the visit.
- Understand that your emotional response to a place is a valid element of the decision-making process.

Glossary

Definitions were often enhanced through the use of the American Heritage Dictionary.

Admission Interview: *The first interview and initial nursing assessment done with you or your loved one upon admission to a care facility. A medical history may be taken. All legal documents required by the facility and by law must also be completed.*

Adult Day Care: *Centers in many communities provide activities — both social and therapeutic — under supervision for aging individuals unable to stay alone during the day. These facilities also have nursing professionals able to monitor your or your loved one's medical needs.*

Advocate: *Although, in our society, attorneys are sometimes called advocates, we use this term to define the person or persons who are speaking up for your loved one's needs and who monitor the care he or she receives. It could be you, it could be the center's Family or Resident Council or it could be the facility's staff.*

Alzheimer's Disease: *A disease marked by progressive loss of mental capacity resulting from degeneration of the brain cells.*

Assisted Living: *This can be a housing option for people who are able to partially care for themselves. Assisted living facilities may offer housekeeping, shopping or transportation help as well as having 24 hour supervision by a care attendant. However, not all assisted living facilities will have staff on duty 24 hours a day. Residences may also offer hair care, bathing help, laundry, in-room meals, etc.*

Beneficiary: *In the legal sense, the recipient of funds, property or other benefits from an insurance policy or will or other legal conveyance.*

Care Conference: *Established by law, care conferences are scheduled regularly to evaluate a resident's care, needs and past and future treatment. Representatives from various departments involved in the care of the resident will attend and provide updates on the current status as it relates to their department. Residents may attend if they desire. Families should attend to ask questions and gather information about their loved one's care.*

Care facility/center: *For the purposes of this handbook, a care facility is one in which residents may receive rehabilitation services or long term (and, if needed, intensive), health care.*

Case Mix: *This refers to the method that many states use to determine nursing home rates for all residents. The case mix is the level of care needed by you or your loved one and is established at least semi-annually by assessments held upon admission to a care facility or a hospital. Included in the assessment are activity of daily living levels, nursing needs or behavioral needs.*

Conservatorship: *A legally defined management arrangement in which one person is responsible for the person and property of another who is incapable of caring for himself or herself.*

Dementia: *Deterioration of intellectual faculties, such as memory, concentration and judgment, resulting from an organic disease or disorder of the brain. It is often accompanied by emotional mood swings and personality changes.*

Discharge Planner: *The person at a hospital responsible for assisting patients and their families in the placement of the patient in other care facilities or rehabilitation programs. This person is often a social worker but may be a nurse or administrator as well.*

Durable Power of Attorney: *This is power of attorney which continues to be valid even after the principal becomes legally incompetent.*

Emergency Measures: *Although the definition of this term will vary, it is generally those medical procedures which will be followed in case of, for example, cardiac or pulmonary arrest. It is VERY important that the care facility clearly define its procedures for you, and it should also make clear what is expected of them by law.*

Family Council: *A group of family members associated with a specific care facility or program. Also called Advocacy Councils. Activities and effectiveness are often determined by the support level of both the families and the facility. The Family Council may support other family members caring for an aged loved one, work with administration to improve and enhance the quality of life for residents and be proactive politically with potential legislative changes which may affect the quality of care for facility residents.*

For profit: *Care centers which operate as for profit business entities are in business to make a profit. They are often privately or publicly held corporations.*

Foster Care: *Adult foster care can take many forms. We define it here as the home which houses aging adults on a long term basis. Foster care facilities are often private homes and deal with fewer residents at a time. Corporations may also sponsor adult foster care homes which are supervised by staff rather than a family.*

Grantor: *A person who creates and funds a trust.*

Incontinent: *A person who lacks normal voluntary control of their excretory functions.*

Irrevocable trust: *A trust which cannot be changed or altered in any way after it is signed.*

Joint Accounts: *These bank accounts may take several forms including joint tenancy, authorized signer or "in trust for" account.*

Living Will: *A legal document which outlines an individual's wishes regarding care in the event of terminal illness or any other drastic change in their physical health. It may indicate the level of heroic measures to be taken in the event of a medical emergency.*

Living Trust: *A trust created during the grantor's lifetime.*

Long Term Care Insurance: *Insurance purchased from a private insurance carrier which is established to help cover the costs of long term care for the individual covered by the policy.*

Medical Assistance: *A program that pays the cost of medical care if a person's assets are at or below established limits. Used interchangeably with the term "Medicaid."*

Medicare: *A program under the US Social Security Administration which reimburses hospitals, some care facilities and physicians for medical care provided to qualifying people over 65 years of age provided the patient meets the qualifying criteria.*

Medicaid: *A program jointly funded by the federal and state governments of the US which reimburses hospitals, some care facilities and physicians for providing care to qualifying people who cannot finance their own medical expenses. Used interchangeably with the term "Medical Assistance."*

Non-profit: *Institutions which do not have monetary gain as their goal and operate their businesses on a break-even basis. Excess revenues are returned to the operations of the institution. In the health care industry, these are often facilities which are affiliated with a philanthropic, service or religious group.*

Nurse's Aide: *A trained assistant who attends to the needs of care facility residents. Federal regulations require these individuals to meet certain licensing requirements.*

Nurse Manager: *Often, the senior nurse on duty of any shift who supervises the activities of the staff and the care needs of the residents or patients. Nurse managers are usually Registered Nurses.*

Nurse Practitioner: *A Registered Nurse with special training for providing primary health care including many tasks customarily performed by a physician.*

Ombudsman for Aging: *Every state is required by the Older Americans Act of 1975 to have an office which resolves complaints or advocates on behalf of nursing home residents. A complete list of these offices follows in Chapter Ten.*

Occupational therapy: *The use of productive or creative activity in the treatment or rehabilitation of physically or emotionally disabled people. Activities may include exploration of new ways for a person to feed or dress themselves or other helpful devices which can increase an individual's sense of dignity. A physician must order the kind, frequency and duration of the treatment.*

Physical therapy: *The treatment of physical dysfunction or injury by the use of therapeutic exercise and other treatments to restore function to the damaged area. A physician must order the kind, frequency and duration of the treatment.*

Power of Attorney: *A legal instrument which authorizes someone to act as another's attorney or agent.*

Recuperation: *The return to full health or strength.*

Rehabilitation: *The restoration of good health, operation or capacity.*

Resident Council: *A group of facility residents which meets regularly to advocate for all the residents of the facility and to communicate concerns to the staff and administration.*

Respite Care: *Assistance provided by individuals who provide caregiving families a break in the responsibility of caring for their loved one. Respite care can be done in the home but facilities often offer short term respite care while families are vacationing or just need a break. There are often relaxed paperwork requirements for respite care admissions to a care center.*

Retirement Center: *For our purposes, a retirement center differs significantly from a long term care facility in that residents may be in excellent health but are looking for a more comfortable, less demanding living environment. Centers may also include other care options of which residents can take advantage if their care needs change drastically.*

Revocable Trust: *A revocable trust can be changed by the grantor at any time as long as he or she is still considered competent.*

Social Activities: *Activities sponsored or implemented by the care facility which offer the residents opportunities to interact with others in a social setting. This category would also include worship services.*

Social Security: *A Federal program that provides economic support to a person faced with unemployment, disability or aging, which is financed by assessment of employees and their employers.*

Social Worker: *A person whose work is intended to advance the social needs of a community through psychological counseling, guidance and assistance.*

Support Group: *A group of individuals, formally or informally organized, which meets regularly to discuss the emotional and psychological needs of its members. By sharing these concerns, the group responds to the needs of its members through compassionate and sympathetic understanding.*

Trusts: *A legal instrument in which a person or financial institution holds legal title and manages assets for the benefit of another person.*

Will: *A legal document which outlines the distribution of a person's estate.*

Resource Information

Offices of the Ombudsmen for the Aging

Alabama
Commission on Aging
770 Washington Avenue
RSA Plaza, Suite 470
Montgomery, AL 36130
334-242-5743
Fax: 334-242-5594

Alaska
Older Alaskans Commission
3601 C Street, Suite 260
Anchorage, AK 99503-5209
907-563-6393
Fax: 907-562-3040

Arizona
Aging and Adult Administration
1789 West Jefferson
Phoenix, AZ 85007
602-542-4446
Fax: 602-542-6575

Arkansas
Department of Human Services
PO Box 1437, Slot 1412
Little Rock, AR 72203-1437
501-682-2441
Fax: 501-682-8155

California
Department of Aging
1600 K Street
Sacramento, CA 95814
916-323-6681
Fax: 916-323-7299

Colorado
The Legal Center
455 Sherman Street, Suite 130
Denver, CO 80203
303-722-0300
Fax: 303-722-0720

Connecticut
Department of Social Services
Elderly Services Division
25 Sigourney Street, 10th Floor
Hartford, CT 06106-5033
203-424-5242
Fax: 203-424-4966

Delaware
Health and Social Services
256 Chapman Road
Oxford Building, Suite 200
Newark, DE 19702
302-453-3820
Fax: 302-453-3836

District of Columbia
AARP, Legal Counsel
for the Elderly
601 E Street NW,
4th Fl., Bldg. A
Washington, D.C. 20049
202-662-4933
Fax: 202-434-6464

Florida
Office of the Governor
Carlton Building
501 South Calhoun Street
Tallahassee, FL 32399-0001
904-488-2039
Fax: 904-488-5657

Georgia
Division of Aging Services
2 Peachtree Street NW, 18th Floor
Atlanta, GA 30303
404-657-5319
Fax: 404-657-5285

Hawaii
Office of the Governor
Executive Office on Aging
335 Merchant Street, Room 241
Honolulu, HI 96813
808-586-0100
Fax: 808-586-0185

Idaho
Commission on Aging
PO Box 83720
Boise, ID 83720-0007
208-334-2220
Fax: 208-334-3033

Illinois
Department on Aging
421 East Capitol Avenue,
No. 100
Springfield, IL 62701
217-785-3140
Fax: 217-785-4477

Indiana
Division of Aging and
Rehabilitation Services
PO Box 7083
402 W. Washington Street,
No. W-454
Indianapolis, IN 46207-7083
317-232-7134
Fax: 317-232-7867

Iowa
Department of Elder Affairs
914 Grand Avenue, No. 236
Jewett Building
Des Moines, IA 50319
515-281-5187
Fax: 515-281-4036

Kansas
Department on Aging
915 SW Harrison
Topeka, KS 66612-1500
913-296-4986
Fax: 913-296-0256

Kentucky
Division of Aging Services
275 E. Main Street, 5th Fl. W
Frankfort, KY 40621
502-564-6930
Fax: 502-564-4595

Louisiana
Governor's Office
of Elderly Affairs
4550 North Blvd. D, 2nd Floor
Baton Rouge, LA 70806
504-925-1700
Fax: 504-925-1749

Maine
160 Capitol Street
PO Box 2723
Augusta, ME 04338-2723
207-621-1079
Fax: 207-621-0509

Maryland
Office of Aging
301 W. Preston Street,
Room 1004
Baltimore, MD 21201
410-225-1100
Fax: 410-333-7943

Massachusetts
Executive Office of Elder Affairs
1 Ashburton Place, 5th Floor
Boston, MA 02108-1518
617-727-7750
Fax: 617-727-9368

Michigan
Citizens for Better Care
416 N. Homer Street, Suite 101
Lansing, MI 48912-4700
517-336-6753

Minnesota
Office of the Ombudsman
on Aging
444 Lafayette Road, 4th Floor
St. Paul, MN 55155-3843
612-296-0382
Fax: 612-297-7855

Mississippi
Division Of Aging and
Adult Services
750 North State Street
Jackson, MS 39202
601-359-4929
Fax: 601-359-4370

Missouri
Division of Aging
Department of Social Services
PO Box 1337
Jefferson City, MO 65102
314-751-3082
Fax: 314-751-8687

Montana
Office on Aging
Department of Family Services
PO Box 8005
Helena, MT 59604-8005
406-444-5900
Fax: 406-444-7743

Nebraska
Department on Aging
301 Centennial Mall South
PO Box 95044
Lincoln, NE 68509-5044
402-471-2306
Fax: 402-471-4619

Nevada
Compliance Investigator
Department of Human Resources
340 N. 11th Street, Suite 203
Las Vegas, NV 89101
702-486-3545
Fax: 702-486-4643

New Hampshire
Division of Elderly and
Adult Services
115 Pleasant Street Annex, Bldg. 1
Concord, NH 03301-3843
603-271-4375
Fax: 603-271-4643

New Jersey
101 South Broad Street
CN808, 7th Floor
Trenton, NJ 08625-0808
609-292-8016
Fax: 609-633-6609

New Mexico
Agency on Aging
228 East Palace Avenue
Santa Fe, NM 87501
505-827-7640
Fax: 505-827-7649

New York
Office for the Aging
Agency Bldg. 42
2 Empire State Plaza
Albany, NY 12223-0001
518-474-0108
Fax: 518-474-0608

North Carolina
Division on Aging
693 Palmer Drive
Raleigh, NC 27603
919-733-3983
Fax: 919-733-0443

North Dakota
Department of Human Services
Aging Service Division
1929 N. Washington
PO Box 58507-7070
Bismarck, ND 58501
701-328-2577
Fax: 701-328-5466

Ohio
Department of Aging
50 W. Broad Street, 9th Floor
Columbus, OH 43215-5928
614-466-1221
Fax: 614-466-5741

Oklahoma
Department of Human Services
Aging Services Division
312 NE 28th Street
Oklahoma City, OK 73105
405-521-6734
Fax: 405-521-2086

Oregon
Office of the Ombudsman on Aging
2475 Lancaster Drive NE, #B-9
Salem, OR 97310
503-378-6533
Fax: 503-3737-0852

Pennsylvania
Department of Aging
400 Market Street, 6th Floor
Harrisburg, PA 17101-2301
717-783-7247
Fax: 717-783-6842

Rhode Island
Department of Elderly Affairs
160 Pine Street
Providence, RI 02903-3708
401-277-2858
Fax: 401-277-2130

South Carolina
Office of the Governor,
Division on Aging
202 Arbor Lane Drive, Suite 301
Columbia, SC 29223-4535
803-737-7500
Fax: 803-737-7501

South Dakota
Office of Adult Services and Aging
Department of Social Services
700 Governors Drive
Pierre, SD 57501-2291
605-773-3656
Fax: 605-773-6834

Tennessee
Regional Ombudsmen Only
For referrals call:
651-741-2056
Fax: 651-741-3309

Texas
Department on Aging
PO Box 12786
Austin, TX 78711
512-444-2727
Fax: 512-440-5252

Utah
Department of Human Services
Division of Aging and
Adult Services
120 North 200 West, Room 401
Salt Lake City, UT 84103
801-538-3924
Fax: 801-538-4395

Vermont
Ombudsman Project
18 Main Street
St. Johnsbury, VT 05819
802-225-2271
Fax: 802-748-4612

Virginia
Department for the Aging
700 East Franklin Street,
10th Floor
Richmond, VA 23219-2327
804-748-8721
Fax: 804-371-8381

Washington
S. King County
Multi-Service Center
1200 South 336th Street
Federal Way, WA 98003-7452
206-838-6810
Fax: 206-874-7831

West Virginia
Commission on Aging
1900 Kanawha Blvd. East
Charleston, WV 25303-0160
304-558-3317
Fax: 304-558-0004

Wisconsin
Board on Aging and
Long Term Care
214 North Hamilton Street
Madison, WI 53703-2118
608-266-8944
Fax: 608-261-6570

Wyoming
Senior Citizens, Inc.
756 Gilchrist
PO Box 94
Wheatland, WY 82201
307-322-5553
Fax: 307-322-3419

Social Security and Medicare
Social Security Administration
1-800-772-1213

Medicare Hotline
1-800-638-6833

National Eldercare Locater Line
For referral services in any state
1-800-677-1116

You may also find assistance from the state and local chapters of the following agencies, senior citizen groups and associations:

American Association of Retired Persons (AARP)
1-202-434-2277

Alzheimer's Association
1-800-438-4380
and from…

- Arthritis Foundation
- American Lung Association
- American Heart Association
- American Diabetes Association
- American Parkinson's Disease Association
- The Multiple Sclerosis Society
- The Society for the Blind
- The Veteran's Administration

Facilities and Alternative Care

American Association of Homes and Services for the Aging
901 E Street NW, Suite 500
Washington, DC 20004-2242
202-783-2242
Fax: 202-783-2255

According to their own literature, the **Continuing Care Accreditation Commission** (CCAC), is the nation's only accrediting commission for non-profit and for-profit continuing care retirement communities. The CCAC's accreditation program is based on the belief that accreditation promotes and maintains quality and integrity in the continuing care industry.

901 E Street NW, Suite 500
Washington, D.C. 20004-2037
202-783-7286
Fax: 202-783-2255

National Council on Aging
408 E Street NW, Second Floor
Washington, DC 20009
202-479-1200

National Hospice Organization
1901 N Fort Myer Drive,
Suite 902
Arlington, VA 22209
703-243-5900

National Citizen's Coalition for Nursing Home Reform
1424 16th Street NW,
Suite 202
Washington, D.C. 20036-2211
202-332-2275
Fax: 202-332-2949

US Department of Health and Human Services
Health Care Financing Administration
200 Independence Avenue SW,
Room 428H
Washington, DC 20201
202-690-6145

Epilogue

On November 8, 1995, Evelyn Marie Mathilda Peterson Schroeder passed from her physical world into her spiritual one. There, she joined her husband of 50 years.

That night we saw a shooting star. We believe to this day that she had finally reunited with him and found the home she had been seeking.

Though Mom never liked any place that took her independence away — living with sons included, the care facilities she lived in were blessed with staffs that worked tirelessly to make her — and her family — comfortable. For that, we, as a family, are deeply grateful. Everyone, from health care professionals to volunteers to the administrators and boards of directors of the facilities, made it possible for Mom to be cared for in a manner which she and her family could find satisfactory.

May your journey include smiles and fond memories and days of peace. It is our sincere hope that the facility you find to meet your needs provides you or your loved one with respect and dignity and treats your family like members of the team.

Acknowledgments

This project was born in our hearts but brought to completion by the help of dozens of people who gave us their support through sharing of their time and thoughts. Our sincere thanks to Robert L. Johnson, Karen Gilgenbach, Linda Lund, Sherilyn Moe, The Rev. William Kaseman, Morrie Lapidos, Michael Sisco, Dr. Robert L. Kane, Kenneth Moritz, John R. Dewey, Lynn Amon, Richard Gehring, Elmer A. Frykman, Ken Covington, Ellie Lundblad, John Jackson and Warren Wolfe.

From the beginning, dedicated friends not only served as our own custom-made support group but also as a cadre of experts who helped us research the industry and create the best document possible. With affection and sincere appreciation, we acknowledge Malcolm McLean, Nadine DeMars, Dr. Kay Schwebke, Don Lehr, Jane Blanco, David Senness, David W. Johnson, Diane Sorensen, Pat Vincent, Rick Moe and Ed Bock. The logistics of production were also in the able hands of friends and family: Starr Morgan and her design firm, Morgan Williams & Associates, and Alan Parker of Parker Printing.

With our abiding love, we thank Don and Joan Schroeder, Lori and Alan, Jodi and Larry, Kristi, Dirk and Lu; Bill and Meg Tuttle, Tony, Danny and Connie, Nathan, Phill, Samantha and Andrew; and Harold and Dorothy Peterson and their family. Without our families, there would be no handbook. Indeed, there would be no story.

We are grateful for the opportunity to share our journey.